This journal is for:

_____

Born:

_____

With all my Love:

_____

Letters to my little boy

Letters to my little boy

Letters to my little boy

Letters to my little boy

Letters to my little boy

Letters to my little boy

Letters to my little boy

Letters to my little boy

Letters to my little boy

Letters to my little boy

Letters to my little boy

Letters to my little boy

Letters to my little boy

Letters to my little boy

Letters to my little boy

Letters to my little boy

Letters to my little boy

Letters to my little boy

Letters to my little boy

Letters to my little boy

Letters to my little boy

Letters to my little boy

Letters to my little boy

Letters to my little boy

Letters to my little boy

Letters to my little boy

Letters to my little boy

Letters to my little boy

Letters to my little boy

Letters to my little boy

Letters to my little boy

Letters to my little boy

Letters to my little boy

 # Letters to my little boy

Letters to my little boy

Letters to my little boy

Letters to my little boy

Letters to my little boy

Letters to my little boy

Letters to my little boy

Letters to my little boy

Letters to my little boy

Letters to my little boy

Letters to my little boy

Letters to my little boy

Letters to my little boy

Letters to my little boy

Letters to my little boy

Letters to my little boy

Letters to my little boy

Letters to my little boy

Letters to my little boy

Letters to my little boy

Letters to my little boy

 # Letters to my little boy

Letters to my little boy

Letters to my little boy

Letters to my little boy

Letters to my little boy

Letters to my little boy

Letters to my little boy

Letters to my little boy

Letters to my little boy

Letters to my little boy

Letters to my little boy

Letters to my little boy

Letters to my little boy

Letters to my little boy

Letters to my little boy

Letters to my little boy

Letters to my little boy

Letters to my little boy

Letters to my little boy

Letters to my little boy

Letters to my little boy

Letters to my little boy

Letters to my little boy

Letters to my little boy

Letters to my little boy

Letters to my little boy

 # Letters to my little boy

Letters to my little boy

Letters to my little boy

Letters to my little boy

Letters to my little boy

Letters to my little boy

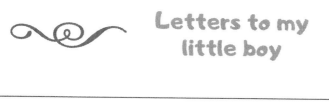

Letters to my little boy

 # Letters to my little boy

Letters to my little boy

Letters to my little boy

Letters to my little boy

Letters to my little boy

Letters to my little boy

Letters to my little boy

Letters to my little boy

Letters to my little boy

Letters to my little boy

 # Letters to my little boy

Letters to my little boy

Letters to my little boy

Letters to my little boy

Letters to my little boy

Letters to my little boy

 # Letters to my little boy

Letters to my little boy

Letters to my little boy

Letters to my little boy

Printed in Great Britain
by Amazon